Ambulance Care Clinical Skills:

Supplementary Checklists

Richard Pilbery
and
Kris Lethbridge

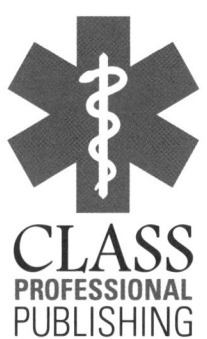

CLASS
PROFESSIONAL
PUBLISHING

Class Professional Publishing have made every effort to ensure that the information, tables, drawings and diagrams contained in this book are accurate at the time of publication. The book cannot always contain all the information necessary for determining appropriate care and cannot address all individual situations; therefore, individuals using the book must ensure they have the appropriate knowledge and skills to enable suitable interpretation. Class Professional Publishing do not guarantee, and accept no legal liability of whatever nature arising from, or connected to, the accuracy, reliability, currency or completeness of the content of *Ambulance Care Clinical Skills: Supplementary Checklists*. Users must always be aware that such innovations or alterations after the date of publication may not be incorporated in the content. Please note, however, that Class Professional Publishing assume no responsibility whatsoever for the content of external resources in the text or accompanying online materials.

Text © Richard Pilbery and Kris Lethbridge 2025

All rights reserved. Without limiting the rights under copyright reserved above, no part of this publication may be reproduced, stored in or introduced into a retrieval system, or transmitted, in any form or by any means (electronic, mechanical, photocopying, recording or otherwise) without the prior written permission of the publisher of this book.

The information presented in this book is accurate and current to the best of the authors' knowledge.

The authors and publisher, however, make no guarantee as to, and assume no responsibility for, the correctness, sufficiency or completeness of such information or recommendation.

Printing history
First published in 2025.
The authors and publisher welcome feedback from the users of this book.

Please contact the publisher:

Class Professional Publishing,
The Exchange, Express Park, Bristol Road, Bridgwater TA6 4RR
Telephone: 01278 472 800
Email: info@class.co.uk
Website: www.classprofessional.co.uk

Class Professional Publishing is an imprint of Class Publishing Ltd
A CIP catalogue record for this book is available from the British Library

Paperback ISBN: 9781801611831
Ambulance Care Clinical Skills and Supplementary Checklists Bundle ISBN: 9781801611848

Cover design by Nicky Borowiec
Designed and typeset by PHi Business Solutions
Printed in the UK by Zenith Print and Packaging

This product is made of material from well-managed forests and other controlled sources. Refer to local recycling guidance on disposal of this book.

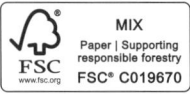

Product safety information can be found at https://www.classprofessional.co.uk/terms-of-use/gpsr-statement/

Contents

Introduction	vii
Patient Assessment	**1**
Respiratory Rate Measurement	1
Record a Peak Flow	3
Record Oxygen Saturations with Pulse Oximetry	5
Record a Pulse	7
Capillary Refill Time Measurement	9
Manual Blood Pressure Measurement	11
Automated Blood Pressure Measurement	13
Record a 3-lead ECG	15
Record a 12-lead ECG	17
Assessing Level of Consciousness with the AVPU Scale	19
Glasgow Coma Scale Score Measurement	21
Face, Arm, Speech, Time Test	23
Blood Sugar Measurement	25
Axillary Temperature Measurement	27
Tympanic Temperature Measurement	29
Airway	**31**
Recovery Position	31
Head Tilt-Chin Lift	33
Jaw Thrust	35
Triple Airway Manoeuvre	37
BURP Manoeuvre	39
Bimanual Laryngoscopy with External Laryngeal Manipulation	41
Airway Foreign-Body Removal with Laryngoscopy	43
Suctioning with a Rigid Suction Catheter	45
Suctioning with a Flexible Suction Catheter	47
Oropharyngeal Airway Insertion	49
Nasopharyngeal Airway Insertion	51
i-gel® Supraglottic Airway Device Insertion	53
Tracheal Intubation	55
Needle Cricothyroidotomy	57
Scalpel Cricothyroidotomy	59
Breathing	**61**
Single-Handed Bag-Valve-Mask Ventilation	61
Two-Handed Bag-Valve-Mask Ventilation	63
Bag-Valve-Mask Ventilation with Positive End-Expiratory Pressure	65
Needle Thoracentesis (Cannula Method)	67
Needle Thoracentesis (PneumoDart Method)	69
Finger Thoracostomy in Adults	71

Contents

Circulation 73
Nasal Clip 73
Modular Bandage 75
Blast® Bandage 77
Haemostatic Dressing – HemCon ChitoGauze® XR Pro 79
Combat Application Tourniquet 81
SOF® Tourniquet 83
Intravenous Cannulation 85
External Jugular Vein Cannulation 87
Intraosseous Access (EZ-IO®) 89

Drug Administration 91
Penthrox® (Methoxyflurane) 91
Spacer Device 93
Inhalers 95
Infusion 97
Drawing Up an Ampoule 99
Oral Administration 101
Nebulising Medication 103
Reconstituting Medications 105
Intramuscular Administration 107
Rectal Administration 109
Intranasal Administration 111

Trauma 113
Broad Arm Sling 113
Elevated Arm Sling 115
Box Splint 117
Vacuum Splint 119
Kendrick Traction Device 121
SAM Pelvic Splint 123
T-POD® Stabilisation Device 125
Manual In-Line Stabilisation 127
Helmet Removal 129
Cervical Collar – Adults 131
Scoop Stretcher 133
Vacuum Mattress 135

Cardiac Arrest 137
Cardiac Arrest: An Advisory Note 137

Infection Prevention and Control 139
Hand Hygiene with Soap and Running Water 139
Hand Hygiene with Alcohol-Based Hand Rub 141
Donning PPE for Standard Infection Prevention Control 143
Donning PPE for Aerosol Generating Procedures 145
Doffing PPE for Standard Infection Prevention Control 147
Doffing PPE for Aerosol Generating Procedures 149

Disclaimer

These checklists are provided for educational and informational purposes only and are intended to support healthcare professionals with training and workflow guidance. They are not designed to diagnose, treat, prevent, or monitor any medical condition.

This product is not classified as a medical device and should be used in conjunction with the *Ambulance Care Clinical Skills* textbook, not as a replacement for professional judgment or clinical decision-making. Paramedics and healthcare professionals should always follow local procedures and be aware of their own scope of practice.

Introduction

The clinical procedures published in *Ambulance Care Clinical Skills* cover a range of practical interventions used by prehospital clinicians. It includes the majority of skills operational ambulance paramedics will require, as well as some skills which may only be relevant to specialist roles. The procedures are based on the latest available evidence and include a detailed rationale for each step. Developing both knowledge of the underpinning theory, as well as competence in the psychomotor skills of procedures relevant to their role is a vital aspect of development for any prehospital provider, regardless of grade. Some skills take many hours to develop, and some can take years of practice to perfect.

Students developing these procedure skills will often have to prepare to be assessed in their practical application, commonly via the form of an Objective Structured Clinical Examination (OSCE). An OSCE is one of many forms of work-based assessment used in modern teaching of health professionals, and normally involve performing the steps of a procedure against a pre-determined standard. Assessors will often use objective pre-defined criteria in the format of checklists, such as those contained in this text, to ensure that all the essential stages of a procedure have been performed as part of the assessment.

The checklists contained within this text do not aim to provide a rationale of actions and do not include every step of every procedure; this is already available in *Ambulance Care Clinical Skills*. Instead, they distil the procedures into a series of short bullet points which can be used as an aide-mémoire when practising or assessing as part of an OSCE assessment. Their use may be particularly valuable as part of peer supported learning where students can assess each other in anticipation of forthcoming OSCEs.

In this first edition we have limited the checklists to those procedures which are easily 'objectively' assessed. Some other more complex procedures, such as advanced life support, have been intentionally omitted on the basis that they are more complex to assess, and training institutions will often use a more complex assessment method rather than a tick box approach to ensure that not only all the essential elements are covered but also that the overall delivery has been appropriate.

The authors would welcome feedback on the use of the checklists, including any additional checklists that may be beneficial for future editions, and we hope you find them useful.

Richard Pilbery
Kris Lethbridge

Patient Assessment

Respiratory Rate Measurement

Action	Check
Don appropriate PPE	
Appropriately position patient so chest is clearly visible	
Count respiratory rate for 1 minute[1]	
Document respiratory rate	

Note:
1. Patients should not be informed that their respiratory rate is being recorded.

Patient Assessment

Record a Peak Flow

Action	Check
Explain procedure to patient	
Obtain consent (unless the patient is unable to)	
Determine patient's normal or best peak flow[1]	
Don appropriate PPE and undertake hand hygiene	
Insert mouthpiece into the peak flow meter	
Ask patient to hold meter with fingers clear of scale and slot	
Ensure holes at end of meter are not blocked	
Check patient position and technique, and adjust if required[2]	
Instruct patient to take a deep breath then blow hard and fast	
Note value on the scale	
Return pointer to zero and repeat procedure twice	
Document highest value from the three readings	

Notes:
1. Patients should be asked if they know what their normal or best peak flow is, or a predicted value chart should be consulted.
2. Patients should be in a standing, or upright sitting, position, and not flex their neck. Patients should hold the meter horizontally, with their fingers clear of the scale and slot.

Patient Assessment

Record Oxygen Saturations with Pulse Oximetry

Action	Check
Explain procedure to patient	
Obtain consent (unless the patient is unable to)	
Don appropriate PPE and undertake hand hygiene	
Ensure device is turned on	
Select appropriate probe and anatomical location[1]	
Connect probe to monitor	
Position probe securely[2]	
Confirm good quality pulse has been detected[3]	
Document findings	

Notes:
1. Measurement errors can occur when probes are used in different anatomical areas or age groups than specified.
2. If possible, avoid arm being used for blood pressure monitoring.
3. Check pulse indicator, waveform and/or perfusion index.

Record a Pulse

Action	Check
Explain procedure to patient	
Obtain consent (unless the patient is unable to)	
Don appropriate PPE and undertake hand hygiene	
Place index and middle fingers along artery and press gently[1]	
Determine the pulse rate[2]	
Document findings	

Notes:
1. General rule for adults is radial pulse first in conscious patient and carotid pulse first in unconscious patient.
2. For regular rhythms, counting for 15 seconds may be appropriate, otherwise count for a full minute.

Patient Assessment

Capillary Refill Time Measurement

Action	Check
Explain procedure to patient/patient's caregiver	
Obtain consent (unless the patient is unable to)	
Don appropriate PPE and undertake hand hygiene	
Check environment is warm and well lit	
Choose appropriate site for measurement[1]	
Apply sufficient pressure for 5 seconds[2]	
Remove pressure and count time for skin to return to normal colour[3]	
Document findings[4]	

Notes:
1. Typically sternum or fingertip.
2. Sufficient pressure can be determined visually, since it will make the tip of clinician's nail blanch.
3. Consider repeating the measurement and averaging the results.
4. A CRT of more than 3 seconds in a child is clinically important.

Patient Assessment

Manual Blood Pressure Measurement

Action	Check
Explain procedure to patient	
Obtain consent (unless the patient is unable to)	
Don appropriate PPE and undertake hand hygiene	
Check patient position	
Choose appropriate arm for measurement	
Palpate brachial artery	
Select correctly sized cuff[1]	
Apply cuff to patient's arm	
Ask patient to remain still and not talk during BP measurement	
Inflate cuff while palpating brachial artery	
Slowly deflate cuff and note return of pulse	
Wait 30 seconds	
Place stethoscope diaphragm over brachial artery	
Inflate cuff	
Deflate cuff noting Korotkoff sounds[2]	
Document blood pressure	

Notes:
1. Using a cuff that is too small will result in an artificially elevated BP reading, and using a cuff that is too large will result in a reading that is artificially low.
2. Note the pressure at which you first hear the Korotkoff sounds (phase 1, the systolic BP), the point at which they become muffled (phase 4) and then disappear (phase 5). The disappearance of sounds is usually taken to be the diastolic BP. If phase 5 continues to 0 mmHg, then the phase 4 measurement should be taken as the diastolic reading.

Patient Assessment

Automated Blood Pressure Measurement

Action	Check
Explain procedure to patient	
Obtain consent (unless the patient is unable to)	
Don appropriate PPE and undertake hand hygiene	
Check patient position	
Choose appropriate arm for measurement	
Select correctly sized cuff[1]	
Connect cuff to monitor	
Apply cuff to patient's arm	
Check correct inflation setting selected	
Ask patient to remain still and not talk during measurement	
Press appropriate button to measure BP	
Document blood pressure	

Note:
1. Using a cuff that is too small will result in an artificially elevated BP reading, and using a cuff that is too large will result in a reading that is artificially low.

Patient Assessment

Record a 3-lead ECG

Action	Check
Explain procedure to patient	
Obtain consent (unless the patient is unable to)	
Don appropriate PPE and undertake hand hygiene	
Position patient	
Expose patient as needed[1]	
Prepare patient's skin	
Check electrodes and attach leads	
Correctly apply limb leads	
Record a 3-lead ECG	
Document procedure and label ECG	

Note:
1. Be mindful of maintaining the patient's dignity and preventing heat loss.

Patient Assessment

Record a 12-lead ECG

Action	Check
Explain procedure to patient	
Obtain consent (unless the patient is unable to)	
Don appropriate PPE and undertake hand hygiene	
Position patient	
Expose patient as needed[1]	
Prepare patient's skin	
Check electrodes and attach leads	
Correctly apply limb leads	
Record a 3-lead ECG	
Document procedure and label ECG	
Prepare chest skin if not already done	
Identify chest landmarks and place V1 and V2	
Place lead V4	
Place lead V3	
Place lead V6	
Place lead V5	
Connect chest lead cables to monitor	
Record 12-lead ECG and check quality	
Document procedure and label ECG	

Note:
1. Be mindful of maintaining the patient's dignity and preventing heat loss.

Patient Assessment

Assessing Level of Consciousness with the AVPU Scale

Action	Check
Explain procedure to patient	
Obtain consent (unless the patient is unable to)	
Don appropriate PPE and undertake hand hygiene	
Observe patient, note any spontaneous behaviours[1]	
Ask patient their name, where they are and what month it is	
Apply pain stimulus if patient unresponsive to voice/being shaken	
Document procedure	

Note:
1. Remember additional category of 'C' for confusion if assessing level of consciousness for NEWS2.

Patient Assessment

Glasgow Coma Scale Score Measurement

Action	Check
Explain procedure to patient	
Obtain consent (unless the patient is unable to)	
Don appropriate PPE and undertake hand hygiene	
Check for factors that might affect assessment[1]	
Observe patient, noting any spontaneous behaviours	
If eye-opening not spontaneous, use verbal stimulus	
If no response to sound, apply central pain stimulus	
Assess verbal response	
Test motor response with two-step action	
If no response to two-step action command, apply central pain stimulus[2]	
Document procedure[3]	

Notes:
1. Includes inability to speak or understand clinician's language, hearing impairments or eye swelling.
2. If there are different responses to left and right sides, record the 'best' response (the response with the higher score).
3. Document each component as well as the total score.

Patient Assessment

Face, Arm, Speech, Time Test

Action	Check
Explain procedure to patient	
Obtain consent (unless the patient is unable to)	
Don appropriate PPE and undertake hand hygiene	
Ask patient to smile or show their teeth	
Lift patient's arms and ask them to hold for 5 seconds[1]	
Check for new speech disturbance	
Document procedure	

Note:
1. Arms should be lifted together to 90° (or 45° if lying on their back).

Patient Assessment

Blood Sugar Measurement

Action	Check
Explain procedure to patient	
Obtain consent (unless the patient is unable to)	
Don appropriate PPE and undertake hand hygiene	
Select appropriate site	
Clean and dry site	
Check use-by date of test strip container	
Insert strip into meter	
Ask patient to dangle arm	
Prick target area with lancet	
After 2 seconds, gently squeeze finger to assist flow of blood	
Touch blood drop to test strip	
Ask patient to apply pressure to puncture site	
Document procedure[1]	

Note:
1. Check the blood sugar result is in the correct units (mmol/l).

Patient Assessment

Axillary Temperature Measurement

Action	Check
Explain procedure to patient	
Obtain consent (unless the patient is unable to)	
Don appropriate PPE and undertake hand hygiene	
Prepare thermometer for use	
Place tip of thermometer high in axilla	
Adduct the patient's arm	
Wait for audible beep	
Remove from axilla and read temperature	
Document procedure[1]	

Note:
1. Check the temperature is recorded in degrees Celsius.

Tympanic Temperature Measurement

Action	Check
Explain procedure to patient	
Obtain consent (unless the patient is unable to)	
Don appropriate PPE and undertake hand hygiene	
Prepare thermometer for use	
Place probe into patient's ear and advance	
Push button that measures temperature	
Wait for thermometer to complete reading	
Remove from ear and read the temperature	
Document procedure[1]	

Note:
1. Check the temperature is recorded in degrees Celsius.

Recovery Position

Action	Check
Don appropriate PPE and undertake hand hygiene	
Kneel beside the patient and straighten both their legs[1]	
Place arm closest to rescuer at right angles to patient's body	
Bring other arm across chest and hold against cheek	
Lift furthest leg at knee ensuring it bends and foot stays on floor	
Roll patient to face rescuer	
Adjust upper leg	
Tilt head to ensure open airway	
Document procedure	

Note:
1. Check pockets for any sharp items that could cause injury on rolling.

Airway

Head Tilt-Chin Lift

Action	Check
Don appropriate PPE and undertake hand hygiene	
Position patient supine	
Place closest hand on patient's head	
Gently tilt head backwards	
Use two fingers to gently lift chin upwards[1]	
Use look, listen, feel to check procedure success	
Document procedure	

Note:
1. Take care not to overextend the neck.

Airway

Jaw Thrust

Action	Check
Don appropriate PPE and undertake hand hygiene	
Position patient supine	
Identify angle of the mandible	
Lift mandible upwards and forwards	
Use thumbs to open patient's mouth	
Document procedure	

Airway

Triple Airway Manoeuvre

Action	Check
Don appropriate PPE and undertake hand hygiene	
Position patient supine	
Identify angle of the mandible	
Lift mandible upwards and forwards	
Use thumbs to open patient's mouth	
Tilt the head backwards	
Document procedure	

BURP Manoeuvre

Action	Check
Don appropriate PPE and undertake hand hygiene	
Place thumb, index and middle fingers on patient's thyroid cartilage	
Provide backward, upward, rightward pressure	
Maintain position and steady pressure until instructed to remove	
Document procedure	

Bimanual Laryngoscopy with External Laryngeal Manipulation

Action	Check
Don appropriate PPE and undertake hand hygiene	
Place thumb, index and middle fingers on patient's thyroid cartilage	
Allow intubating clinician to move your hand into optimal position	
Keep pressure and direction applied to larynx	
Remove pressure when instructed by intubating clinician	
Document procedure	

Airway Foreign-Body Removal with Laryngoscopy

Action	Check
Don appropriate PPE and undertake appropriate hand hygiene	
Prepare equipment, to include as a minimum: • Suction • Laryngyscope and blade • Oxygen • Bag-valve-mask • Magill forceps	
Appropriately position patient	
Visually inspect anterior oropharynx	
If FBAO visible, remove with Magill forceps	
Open the airway into the 'sniffing the morning air' position	
Open the mouth and inspect the oral cavity[1]	
Insert laryngoscope into mouth	
Suction, if required	
Advance blade until FBAO observed	
Use Magill forceps to carefully remove FBAO	
Attempt to oxygenate, with ventilations if required	
If unsuccessful, repeat procedure once[2]	
Document procedure	

Notes:
1. If the mouth needs opening further to inspect the oral cavity, the 'scissor' technique should be used.
2. If you cannot remove a FBAO after two attempts, concentrate on providing chest compressions instead.

Airway

Suctioning with a Rigid Suction Catheter

Action	Check
Don appropriate PPE, including respiratory protective equipment (RPE) if suctioning beyond the oropharynx, and undertake appropriate hand hygiene	
Prepare equipment: • Suction unit • Rigid wide-bore and soft-tip catheters and suction tubing • Oxygen	
Appropriately position patient	
Attach suction tubing and catheter and switch on unit	
Open patient's mouth and insert catheter without suctioning[1]	
Apply suction, occluding vent hole if present, while withdrawing catheter	
Re-oxygenate and reassess airway	
Repeat procedure if required[2]	
Document procedure	

Notes:
1. This is not possible with suction catheters that have no vent hole. Take care not to damage soft tissue.
2. If procedure is being performed in a cardiac arrest scenario, then this procedure should be limited to two attempts before moving on to chest compressions.

Airway

Suctioning with a Flexible Suction Catheter

Action	Check
Don appropriate PPE, including respiratory protective equipment (RPE) if suctioning beyond the oropharynx, and undertake appropriate hand hygiene	
Prepare equipment: • Suction unit • Rigid wide-bore and soft-tip catheters and suction tubing • Oxygen	
Explain procedure to the patient and obtain consent where possible	
Appropriately position patient	
Attach suction tubing and catheter and switch on unit	
Keep thumb clear of suction port	
Insert catheter no further than end of airway adjunct or tracheostomy tube	
Apply suction by occluding suction port and gently withdraw catheter	
Re-oxygenate and reassess airway	
Repeat procedure if required	
Document procedure	

Oropharyngeal Airway Insertion

Action	Check
Don appropriate PPE and undertake hand hygiene	
Select correctly sized OPA	
Open patient's mouth and ensure it is clear of foreign bodies	
Insert airway 'upside down' along roof of mouth to soft palate	
Rotate OPA through 180°	
Advance OPA until it rests in the pharynx[1]	
Continue to provide manual manoeuvres	
Document procedure	

Note:
1. A jaw thrust can help seat the OPA in the correct position.

Nasopharyngeal Airway Insertion

Action	Check
Don appropriate PPE and undertake hand hygiene	
Prepare equipment: • Appropriately sized NPA • Water-soluble gel • Suction	
Lubricate NPA	
Insert NPA posteriorly with bevel facing the nasal septum[1]	
Confirm position	
Document procedure	

Note:
1. If the NPA cannot be advanced after gentle twisting, consider changing nostrils or using a smaller size.

i-gel® Supraglottic Airway Device Insertion

Action	Check
Don appropriate PPE and undertake hand hygiene	
Ensure airway is clear	
Prepare equipment: • Oxygen • Suction • Bag-valve-mask • Magill forceps • i-gel® • OPA • 'Airway tree' • Lubricant • i-gel® securing device • Stethoscope	
Select correct size i-gel®	
Open packaging, remove i-gel® from cradle	
Lubricate back, sides and front tip of i-gel®	
Perform laryngoscopy if foreign body suspected	
Appropriately position patient's airway[1]	
Introduce i-gel® into patients mouth	
Glide downwards and backwards until definitive resistance felt	
Connect i-gel® to 'airway tree'	
Secure the device appropriately	
Re-check placement after moving or change in patient condition	
Document procedure	

Note:
1. The patient should be in the 'sniffing the morning air' position.

Tracheal Intubation

Action	Check
Don appropriate PPE and undertake hand hygiene	
Adjust patient position, if required	
Ensure airway is clear and ventilate	
Assistant should prepare: • Oxygen • Suction • Bag-valve-mask • Magill forceps • Laryngoscope • Bougie • OPA • 'Airway tree' • Tracheal tubes • Syringe • Tube securing device • Stethoscope	
Consider whether patient may be difficult to intubate[1]	
Make and communicate intubation plan	
Appropriately position patient's airway[2]	
Open mouth and inspect the oropharynx. Suction as required.	
Utilise checklist to ensure equipment and team are ready	
Gently insert laryngoscope and sweep tongue to left	
Slowly advance blade in the midline until epiglottis visible	
Insert tip of blade into vallecula	
Lift blade at an angle of 45° until posterior/arytenoid cartilages are visible	
Ask assistant to pass the bougie	
Insert bougie into right-side of patient's mouth	
Insert bougie through cords[3]	
Ask assistant to thread tube over bougie	
Communicate tube handover and gently advance through the cords	

Chapter 2 – Airway

Action	Check
Ask assistant to remove bougie	
Ask assistant to inflate the tube cuff	
Attach 'airway tree'	
Confirm placement with end-tidal CO_2 and auscultation	
One placement confirmed, remove laryngoscope	
Secure tube	
Document procedure	

Notes:
1. Use the LEMON mnemonic.
2. The patient should be in the 'sniffing the morning air' position.
3. Once approximately 22–24 cm of the bougie is in the adult patient's mouth, do not advance any further.

Needle Cricothyroidotomy

Action	Check
Don appropriate PPE and undertake hand hygiene	
Communicate intention to undertake procedure with the team	
Prepare equipment: • Large bore cannula • 3-way tap with extension tubing • Oxygen tubing • 10 or 20 ml syringe • Sharps container • Saline flush (optional)	
Attach oxygen tubing to 3-way tap and open ports	
Set oxygen flow rate to 15 l/min	
Extend patient's head/hyperextend the neck	
Appropriately position yourself	
Immobilise the larynx and palpate cricothyroid membrane	
Ask assistant to pass cannula affixed to syringe	
Direct cannula with syringe caudally along axis of trachea at an angle of 30°	
Insert cannula, aspirating the syringe as you advance	
Stop once air can be easily aspirated	
Hold needle and syringe still and advance catheter	
Remove catheter needle and attach port at end of 3-way tap	
Attempt to ventilate[1]	
If possible, hold cannula in position	
Document procedure	

Note:
1. The ventilation ratio is 1 second inspiration to 3 seconds expiration.

Scalpel Cricothyroidotomy

Action	Check
Don appropriate PPE and undertake hand hygiene	
Communicate intention to undertake procedure with the team	
Prepare equipment: • Size 10 scalpel • Size 10 fr bougie • 6 mm cuffed tracheal tube • 10 ml syringe • Tape • Bag-valve-mask • Ventilation circuit • Stethoscope • Gauze	
Appropriately position patient	
Appropriately position yourself	
Identify cricothyroid membrane and anchor cricoid cartilage[1]	
Make horizontal stab incision through centre of cricoid membrane	
Turn blade through 90°	
Ask assistant to pass bougie	
Insert bougie tip along the side of the scalpel and into the trachea	
Remove scalpel	
Ask assistant to place tracheal tube on bougie and slide it down	
Communicate handover of the bougie	
Railroad tube over bougie and into trachea	
Ask assistant to gently remove bougie	
Inflate cuff and gently ventilate	
Confirm placement of tube	
Document procedure	

Chapter 2 – *Airway*

Note:
1. Grasp the patient's trachea between your thumb and index finger, slowly move your fingers up, with your thumb on one side of the trachea and the middle finger on the other side. Use your index finger to palpate the midline, feeling for the cricothyroid membrane. Once identified, use your thumb and middle finger to anchor the cricoid cartilage and the index finger to mark the position of the cricothyroid membrane.

Breathing

Single-Handed Bag-Valve-Mask Ventilation

Action	Check
Don appropriate PPE and undertake hand hygiene	
Open the patient's airway and adjust head position	
Perform visual check of oropharynx	
Ventilating clinician should locate to head of patient	
Assess for signs of ventilation difficulty	
Insert appropriately sized oro- and/or naso-pharyngeal airway(s)	
Select correctly sized mask	
Connect mask to bag, capnography and oxygen supply	
Position mask on patient's face	
Position hands on the mask to keep it in position while lifting the jaw to meet the mask	
Gently squeeze the bag just enough to make the chest rise	
Adjust airway position if ventilation difficult	
Frequently reassess adequacy of ventilation	
Document procedure	

Two-Handed Bag-Valve-Mask Ventilation

Breathing

Action	Check
Don appropriate PPE and undertake hand hygiene	
Open the patient's airway and adjust head position	
Perform visual check of oropharynx	
Ventilating clinician should locate to head of patient	
Assess for signs of ventilation difficulty	
Insert appropriately sized oro- and/or naso-pharyngeal airway(s)	
Select correctly sized mask	
Connect mask to bag, capnography and oxygen supply	
Position mask on patient's face	
Mask-holding clinician: Place both thenar eminences on top of mask with thumbs facing caudally	
Mask-holding clinician: Grasp mandible and pull it forward to meet mask	
Non-mask-holding clinician: Gently squeeze bag just enough to see chest rise	
Adjust airway position if ventilation difficult	
Frequently reassess adequacy of ventilation	
Document procedure	

Breathing

Bag-Valve-Mask Ventilation with Positive End-Expiratory Pressure

Action	Check
Identify need for positive end-expiratory pressure (PEEP) during bag-valve-mask (BVM) ventilation	
Inspect valve for damage	
Remove outlet cap from BVM	
Set correct initial PEEP value	
Attach PEEP valve	
Adjust PEEP as required	
Frequently recheck set level of PEEP	
Document procedure	

Breathing

Needle Thoracentesis (Cannula Method)

Action	Check
Don appropriate PPE and undertake hand hygiene	
Prepare your equipment: • Large-bore cannula • 10 ml syringe • Saline flush • Skin-cleansing wipe • Roll of tape • Chest seal • Sharps container	
Locate correct site	
Clean site and allow to dry	
(Optional) Draw up 3–4 ml of saline into the syringe and attach to cannula	
Insert cannula at 90° to patient's back[1]	
Advance cannula while gently pulling back on plunger	
Once sudden loss of resistance or bubbles in syringe, stop insertion	
Anchor syringe and needle, and advance cannula	
Remove syringe and needle and dispose into sharps container	
Reassess patient	
If unsuccessful, repeat procedure using lateral approach[2]	
Secure cannula	
Document procedure	

Notes:
1. This should be close to the top of the patient's third rib to avoid the neurovascular bundle under the second rib.
2. Fifth intercostal space just anterior to the mid-axillary line.

Needle Thoracentesis (PneumoDart Method)

Action	Check
Don appropriate PPE and undertake hand hygiene	
Prepare your equipment: • PneumoDart • Skin-cleansing wipe • Materials to secure needle • Sharps container	
Locate correct site	
Clean site and allow to dry	
Inspect safety seal on PneumoDart and remove needle from case	
Insert cannula at 90° to the chest wall[1]	
Observe needle position indicator moving backwards	
Advance needle towards patient's back	
Once needle penetrates pleura, note movement of indicator and release of air	
Secure needle in place	
Reassess patient	
Document procedure	

Note:
1. This should be close to the top of the patient's third rib to avoid the neurovascular bundle under the second rib.

Finger Thoracostomy in Adults

Action	Check
Explain procedure and obtain consent (unless the patient is unable to)	
Don appropriate PPE and undertake hand hygiene	
Prepare your equipment: • Size 22 scalpel • ChloraPerp skin prep (or similar) • Spencer Wells forceps • One-way dressing • Sharps container	
Position patient appropriately	
If the patient is conscious, administer analgesia, sedation or local anaesthetic	
Identify triangle of safety	
Clean the area	
Make incision with scalpel[1]	
Dispose of scalpel in sharps container	
Insert Spencer Wells forceps and 'punch through' the intercostal muscle	
Gently rotate and open and close the forceps to enlarge the opening	
Slide index finger into hole while forceps still in situ	
Once finger inside chest cavity remove forceps	
Sweel finger through 360° to palpate lung	
If patient spontaneously breathing place one-way occlusive dressing over hole	
Continually reassess for signs of a tension pneumothorax redeveloping	
Document procedure	

Note:
1. Make an incision in the fifth intercostal space, over the top of the inferior rib between the mid-axillary and the anterior axillary lines. The incision should be approximately 3–5 cm long and deep enough to cut through the skin and underlying fat.

Nasal Clip

Action	Check
Explain the procedure and obtain consent (unless the patient is unable to)	
Don appropriate PPE and undertake hand hygiene	
Adopt first-aid measures	
Prepare the clip	
Pinch the nose with the clip and increase pressure	
If patient starts to bleed from mouth or into oropharynx, consider alternative management	
Release clip after 10–12 minutes and reassess	
Document the procedure	

Circulation

Modular Bandage

Action	Check
If the patient is conscious, explain the procedure and obtain consent (unless the patient is unable to)	
Don appropriate PPE and undertake hand hygiene	
Open outer plastic wrapper and remove dressing	
Ensure wound is ready to be dressed[1]	
Place centre of dressing directly over wound	
Wrap the bandage around the dressing	
Finish the bandage[2]	
Check pulse distal to dressing	
If necessary, apply direct pressure on top of the dressing	
Document the procedure	

Notes:
1. Deep wounds should be packed with gauze or, if necessary, a haemostatic dressing.
2. To finish the bandage, ensure the Velcro on the end of the bandage is stuck down and loop the plastic hooks under one of the previous wraps of material.

Circulation

Blast® Bandage

Action	Check
If the patient is conscious, explain the procedure and obtain consent (unless the patient is unable to)	
Don appropriate PPE and undertake hand hygiene	
Open outer plastic wrapper and remove dressing	
Ensure wound is ready to be dressed[1]	
Gather the end of the amputated limb into the dressing	
Place a single wrap of bandage around dressing to secure it	
Wrap bandage around the end of the dressing	
Finish the bandage[2]	
Check pulse distal to dressing	
If necessary, apply direct pressure on top of the dressing or place another Blast bandage over the top	
Document the procedure	

Notes:
1. For an amputated limb, a tourniquet may need to be applied to gain control of bleeding.
2. To finish the bandage, ensure the Velcro on the end of the bandage is stuck down and loop the plastic hooks under one of the previous wraps of material.

Circulation

Haemostatic Dressing – HemCon ChitoGauze® XR Pro

Action	Check
Explain the procedure and obtain consent (unless the patient is unable to)	
Don appropriate PPE and undertake hand hygiene	
Open package and remove ChitoGauze®	
Pack gauze deep into the wound	
Cut off excess dressing	
Maintain direct pressure until bleeding controlled	
Dress the wound	
Continually reassess wound area and dressing	
Document the procedure	

Circulation

Combat Application Tourniquet

Action	Check
Explain the procedure and obtain consent (unless the patient is unable to)	
Don appropriate PPE and undertake hand hygiene	
Place the tourniquet around the limb and directly on to the skin[1]	
Pull band of material through the buckle	
Once tight, stick it back to itself around the limb	
Turn the rod until the bleeding stops	
Continue turning rod until it can be clipped into holder	
Wrap remaining strap and place time strap over the top to secure the rod	
Document the procedure	
Continually reassess the tourniquet	

Note:
1. Place the tourniquet around the limb, around 5–8 cm (approximately 2–3 in) above the site of bleeding directly on to the skin. This can be on a single- or double-bone limb but should not be immediately over a joint.

Circulation

SOF® Tourniquet

Action	Check
Explain the procedure and obtain consent (unless the patient is unable to)	
Don appropriate PPE and undertake hand hygiene	
Place the tourniquet around the limb and directly on to the skin[1]	
Clip buckle on the strap to the body of the tourniquet	
Stabilise and pull the strap until slack has been taken out	
Turn the rod until the bleeding stops	
Keep turning rod until it can be clipped into holder	
Wrap remaining strap	
Document the procedure	
Continually reassess the tourniquet	

Note:
1. Place the tourniquet around the limb, around 5–8 cm (approximately 2–3 in) above the site of bleeding directly on to the skin. This can be on a single- or double-bone limb but should not be immediately over a joint.

Circulation

Intravenous Cannulation

Action	Check
Explain the procedure and obtain consent (unless the patient is unable to)	
Don appropriate PPE and undertake hand hygiene	
Identify an appropriate site	
Choose an appropriately sized cannula	
Prepare the remainder of your equipment: • Tourniquet • Appropriate skin preparation wipe (as per local policy) • Your selected size cannula and a size smaller • A 10 ml syringe, filled with 0.9% saline or a pre-filled syringe • A sharps bin • A cannula dressing • A dressing/gauze in case the attempt is unsuccessful	
Apply tourniquet	
Thoroughly clean the site	
Anchor the skin around the insertion site with non-dominant hand	
Insert the cannula and watch for flashback	
Once you have flashback, flatten the cannula and advance slightly	
Adjust hand position and gently pull needle back slightly	
Advance plastic cannula	
Remove the tourniquet	
Anchor cannula to skin and occlude tip	
Remove sharp	
Screw cap on back of cannula	
Dispose of sharp in a sharps bin	
Apply dressing strips if present	
Flush the cannula	
Fix cannula with remainder of dressing	
Document the procedure	

Circulation

External Jugular Vein Cannulation

Action	Check
If the patient is conscious, explain the procedure and obtain consent (unless the patient is unable to)	
Don appropriate PPE and undertake hand hygiene	
Lay the patient flat or, if safe, slightly head down	
Identify the external jugular vein	
Choose an appropriately sized cannula	
Prepare the remainder of your equipment: <ul><li>Appropriate skin preparation wipe (as per local policy)</li><li>Your selected size cannula and a size smaller</li><li>A 10 ml syringe, filled with 0.9% saline or a pre-filled syringe</li><li>A sharps bin</li><li>A cannula dressing</li><li>A dressing/gauze in case the attempt is unsuccessful</li></ul>	
Thoroughly clean the site	
Anchor the skin around the insertion site with non-dominant hand	
Insert the cannula and watch for flashback	
Once you have flashback, flatten the cannula and advance	
Adjust hand position and gently pull needle back slightly	
Advance plastic cannula	
Anchor cannula to skin and occlude tip	
Remove sharp	
Screw cap on back of cannula	
Dispose of sharp in a sharps bin	
Apply cannula dressing	
Flush the cannula	
Ensure dressing is secure	
Document the procedure	

Circulation

Intraosseous Access (EZ-IO®)

Action	Check
Explain the procedure and obtain consent (unless the patient is unable to)	
Don appropriate PPE and undertake hand hygiene	
Select most appropriate site	
Gather required equipment: • A skin-cleansing wipe • An appropriately sized needle • The insertion driver • Primed connecting line • 10 ml syringe with sodium chloride for flushing the line • Lidocaine (if conscious) • An appropriate dressing • Sharps bin	
Identify the site	
Choose appropriately sized needle	
Clean the site	
Test the driver	
Attach needle to the end of the driver	
Stabilise the extremity	
Without pulling the trigger, insert needle through skin at 90 degrees	
Check angle of drill is appropriate for penetrating underlying bone	
Check at least one 5mm black marker is visible	
Pull trigger while applying light pressure	
Keep trigger squeezed until needle is pulled into the bone	
Disconnect driver	
Place stabiliser over the needle	
Attach the administration set and flush	
Fix down stabiliser	
Apply wrist band to patient with site and time of insertion recorded	
Document the procedure	

Penthrox® (Methoxyflurane)

Action	Check
Explain the procedure and obtain consent (unless the patient is unable to)	
Don appropriate PPE and undertake hand hygiene	
Open package and check all components	
Attach the activated carbon filter	
Open the vial	
Pour methoxyflurane into the back of the device[1]	
Place wrist loop over the patient's wrist	
Instruct the patient to breathe through the inhaler	
Consider if further analgesia is required	
Once device has been used, dispose of correctly	
Document the procedure	

Note:
1. Tilt the inhaler to a 45° angle with the mouthpiece pointing down. Continually rotate the device while pouring.

Drug Administration

Spacer Device

Action	Check
Explain the procedure and obtain consent (unless the patient is unable to)	
Don appropriate PPE and undertake hand hygiene	
Examine spacer for damage	
Remove cap from pMDI and shake	
Insert pMDI into the back of the chamber	
Explain the required technique to the patient	
Document the procedure	

Drug Administration

Inhalers

Action	Check
Explain the procedure and obtain consent (unless the patient is unable to)	
Don appropriate PPE and undertake hand hygiene	
Inspect inhaler for damage	
Check canister is in date	
Remove cap from end of inhaler and check for foreign bodies	
Shake the inhaler well	
Instruct patient how to grip the inhaler and on correct inhaler technique	
Consider whether further doses are required after 30–60 seconds	
When patient has finished with inhaler, replace cap and store safely	
Document the procedure	

Drug Administration

Infusion

Action	Check
Don appropriate PPE and undertake hand hygiene	
Prepare the required equipment: • The fluid for administration • A giving set	
Check packaging of the giving set	
Examine the fluid	
Remove packaging and hang up fluid	
Twist and remove foil covering or rubber pigtail from the outlet channel	
Open giving set packaging	
Close the roller clamp	
Remove protective cap from end of the spike	
Push spike straight into fluid outlet channel	
Prime the drip chamber	
Gently open the roller clamp until fluid starts to slowly flow through the line	
Inspect the line for air bubbles	
Inspect the drip chamber to ensure it is half-full	
Document the procedure	

Drug Administration

Drawing Up an Ampoule

Action	Check
Don appropriate PPE and undertake appropriate hand hygiene	
Prepare the required equipment: • The ampoule of medication • An appropriately sized syringe • Ampoule breakers • Drawing-up needle • Syringe bung • Drug label (if appropriate) • Sharps bin	
Check the following: • Integrity of the ampoule • The medication is the correct drug and dose • The contents appear as expected • The expiry date is clearly visible and the ampoule is within date	
Ensure all liquid is in the main body of the ampoule	
Place disposable ampoule breaker into position	
Snap the top off the ampoule[1]	
Dispose in a sharps bin	
Inspect the contents for the ampoule for glass fragments	
Attach blunt filter needle (drawing-up needle) to the syringe	
Aspirate fluid from the ampoule into the syringe	
Remove air bubbles, if present	
Remove drawing-up needle and dispose of it safely	
Label and bung syringe if medication not to be used immediately	
Document the procedure	

Note:
1. Ensure dot on the neck of the ampoule is facing away from you.

Oral Administration

Action	Check
Explain the procedure and obtain consent (unless the patient is unable to)	
Don appropriate PPE and undertake appropriate hand hygiene	
Check the medication package: • Integrity of all packaging • Medication is correct drug and dose • Expiry date is visible and drug in date	
Prior to administration, complete a med-check process	
Present medication to patient with clear instructions	
Assist patient appropriately if they cannot administer medication themselves[1]	
Document the procedure	

Note:
1. Do not place tablet into mouth of a patient unless you are confident they can swallow effectively.

Nebulising Medication

Action	Check
Explain the procedure and obtain consent (unless the patient is unable to)	
Don appropriate PPE and undertake appropriate hand hygiene	
Open nebuliser mask packaging	
Prior to administration, complete a med-check	
Add medication to nebuliser chamber	
Connect gas tubing to chamber and seat mask on patient's face	
Turn on gas flow at 8 l/min	
Coach the patient's breathing	
Monitor the administration of nebulised medication	
Document the procedure	

Drug Administration

Reconstituting Medications

Action	Check
Explain the procedure and obtain consent (unless the patient is unable to)	
Don appropriate PPE and undertake appropriate hand hygiene	
Prepare the required equipment: • The ampoule of medication to be prepared • Required quantity of base fluid • Appropriately sized syringe • Blunt filter needle • Sharps bin	
Before commencing, confirm: • The medication • The dose • The type of base fluid	
Draw up correct amount of base fluid	
Take cap off vial for reconstitution	
Place blunt needle through rubber seal and inject base fluid into ampoule	
Mix fluid and drug together	
Invert vial and aspirate contents into syringe	
Once aspirated, inspect contents	
Prior to administration, complete a med-check	
Dispose of ampoule and drawing up needle securely	
Document the procedure	

Drug Administration

Intramuscular Administration

Action	Check
Explain the procedure and obtain consent (unless the patient is unable to)	
Don appropriate PPE and undertake appropriate hand hygiene	
Prepare the required equipment, including: • The appropriate medication • An appropriately sized syringe • A blunt filter drawing-up needle • Sharps bin • Disinfectant wipe • A syringe label (if appropriate) • Gauze • Roll of medical tape • A needle for administering the medication • Plaster	
Follow ampoule drawing-up procedure	
Inspect site for administration	
Thoroughly clean the site	
Prior to administration, complete a med-check process	
Firmly attach needle to syringe and remove cap	
Apple gentle traction to injection site with non-dominant hand	
Warn patient of sharp scratch	
Insert needle at 90 degrees to the skin	
Aspirate the syringe and observe for blood	
Inject fluid at rate of approximately 1ml every 10 seconds	
Remove needle and place in sharps bin	
Release traction and apply pressure with gauze for a few seconds	
Replace the gauze with a small plaster	
Document the procedure	

Drug Administration

Rectal Administration

Action	Check
Explain the procedure and obtain consent (unless the patient is unable to)	
Don appropriate PPE and undertake appropriate hand hygiene	
Ensure a chaperone is present	
Position the patient appropriately	
Inspect the packaging	
Remove cap from end of rectal tube	
Prior to administration, complete a med-check process	
Lift upper buttock to reveal anus	
Insert nozzle completely into rectum[1]	
Empty the tube	
Remove tube and dispose in clinical waste bin	
If possible and safe, maintain the patient in a side or face-down position for a couple of minutes	
Document the procedure	

Note:
1. For children under 15kg, insert nozzle half-way.

Intranasal Administration

Action	Check
Explain the procedure and obtain consent (unless the patient is unable to)	
Don appropriate PPE and undertake appropriate hand hygiene	
Prepare the required equipment: • The appropriate medication • An appropriately sized Luer Lock syringe • A blunt filter drawing-up needle • Sharps bin • A nasal atomiser device • A syringe label (if appropriate)	
Follow the procedure for drawing up an ampoule[1]	
Connect nasal atomiser to syringe	
Prior to administration, complete a med-check process	
Use your free hand to hold the patient's occiput stable	
Place tip of atomiser device snugly against the nostril	
Briskly depress the plunger and deliver half of the medication into one nostril	
Move syringe and nasal atomiser device to other nostril and deliver remaining medication	
Document the procedure	

Note:
1. Only draw up the amount of medication to be administered, plus an additional 0.1ml.

Trauma

Broad Arm Sling

Action	Check
Explain the procedure and obtain consent (unless the patient is unable to)	
Don appropriate PPE and undertake appropriate hand hygiene	
Remove clothing from the injured limb and conduct a full neurovascular assessment	
Dress wounds, if present	
Ensure the patient has adequate analgesia	
Ask the patient to support their injured arm with the uninjured arm and to flex the elbow to 90 degrees	
Open the triangular bandage and gently pass it under the injured arm with the point under the elbow of the injured arm	
Slide the upper end of the triangular bandage around the back of the neck towards the shoulder on the injured side	
Lift the other end of the triangular bandage up over the forearm	
Tie the two ends together, preferably using a reef knot, to the side of the neck. Consider use of padding	
Take hold of the point of the bandage beyond the elbow and twist until the fabric is snug to the elbow. Then fold the excess into the bandage or tape it to the outside	
Recheck the limb distally for any change in neurovascular status	
Document the procedure	

Elevated Arm Sling

Action	Check
Explain the procedure and obtain consent (unless the patient is unable to)	
Don appropriate PPE and undertake appropriate hand hygiene	
Remove clothing from the injured limb and conduct a full neurovascular assessment	
Dress wounds, if present	
Ensure the patient has adequate analgesia	
Ask the patient to support their injured arm with the uninjured arm[1]	
Place the triangular bandage over the injured arm with the point on the bandage just beyond the elbow of the injured arm	
Ask the patient to let go of the injured arm and tuck the bandage under the injured arm and bring it around to their back	
Bring the bandage up across the patients back to meet the other end at the shoulder on the uninjured side	
Tie the two ends together, preferably using a reef knot, to the side of the neck. Consider use of padding	
Take hold of the point of the bandage beyond the elbow and twist until the fabric is snug to the elbow. Then fold the excess into the bandage or tape it to the outside	
Recheck the limb distally for any change in neurovascular status	
Document the procedure	

Note:
1. The injured arm should be placed across their chest with the fingers of the injured arm resting on the opposite shoulder.

Box Splint

Action	Check
Explain the procedure and obtain consent (unless the patient is unable to)	
Don appropriate PPE and undertake appropriate hand hygiene	
Remove clothing from the injured limb and conduct a full neurovascular assessment	
Dress wounds, if present	
Choose an appropriately sized splint	
Ensure the patient has received adequate analgesia	
Open the splint and place it next to, or in line with, the injured limb with the Velcro pointing out towards you. Prepare additional padding, if required	
In a coordinated move with other team members, lift the limb just enough to move the splint into position. Warn the patient in advance	
Once the splint is in position, lower the limb back on to the splint	
Lift the two side pieces to create an open box shape around the limb. Lift foot plate, if present, so it sits against the sole of the foot	
Gently fasten the Velcro straps to the opposite side of the splint, taking care to avoid placing straps directly over the site of the injury	
Consider padding for large gaps around the limb inside the splint	
Recheck distal pulse and sensation	
Document the procedure	

Vacuum Splint

Action	Check
Explain the procedure and obtain consent (unless the patient is unable to)	
Don appropriate PPE and undertake appropriate hand hygiene	
Remove clothing from the injured limb and conduct a full neurovascular assessment	
Dress wounds, if present	
Choose an appropriately sized splint	
Ensure the patient has received adequate analgesia	
Open the splint and place it next to the injured limb with the valve pointing towards you	
Open the valve to allow air to enter and use your hand to evenly distribute the polystyrene ball bearings inside so that the splint is flat	
Securely close the valve	
In a coordinated move with other team members, lift the limb just enough to slip the splint into position. Warn the patient in advance	
Once the splint is in position, lower the limb back on to the splint	
Form the splint around the injured limb[1]	
Attach the pump to the valve and, while the splint is being held in position, another team member operates the pump until the splint becomes firm	
Once the splint is firm, remove the pump	
Wrap the Velcro straps around the splint	
Recheck distal pulse and sensation	
Regularly check the splint during transport	
Document the procedure	

Note:
1. Try to leave the end of the splint open and a small gap of approximately 2.5 cm (1 in) along the top of the splint so the limb can still be visualised. If required, the straps can be loosely placed at this point to help keep the splint in shape.

Kendrick Traction Device

Action	Check
Explain the procedure and obtain consent (unless the patient is unable to)	
Don appropriate PPE and undertake appropriate hand hygiene	
Ensure all the patient's clothing has been removed from the leg	
Ensure that all parts are present	
Apply ankle strap and secure with Velcro	
Place the thigh strap under the back of the knee	
Slide the thigh strap so that it is high in the groin. Ensure genitals are not trapped	
Clip the buckle on the superior aspect of the limb	
Adjust the strap so that the pole receptacle is level with the iliac crest	
Take the pole and straighten it out. Then place it next to the patient and ensure that at least one full section of pole extends below the foot	
Adjust length of pole and insert into receptacle	
Place the yellow strap around the knee and secure	
Place the dart on the end of the black pole through the yellow loop on the section of strap that hangs down from the foot	
Apply traction by simultaneously pulling down on the red tab on the foot strap and feeding the other side of the strap with the yellow tab through the buckle	
Apply until normal anatomical alignment or significant reduction in pain is achieved	
Apply straps over the thigh and ankle	
Assess the pulse, movement and sensation distally on the limb	
Document the procedure	

Trauma

SAM Pelvic Splint

Action	Check
Explain the procedure and obtain consent (unless the patient is unable to)	
Don appropriate PPE and undertake appropriate hand hygiene	
Check all the patient's clothing (including underwear) has been removed	
Choose the correctly sized binder based on patient waist size	
Locate the level of the greater trochanter	
As long as there are no other injuries that may be made worse, strap the feet together using a triangle bandage (or similar) in a figure of eight	
Insert the binder under the legs	
Slide the binder up into position and confirm the centre of the binder is in line with the greater trochanters	
Pull the strap through the orange buckle, and ensure that there is an equal amount of binder on each side of the patient	
With one person on each side, pull the black strap and orange handle in opposite directions until the buckle clicks	
Maintain tension and secure the Velcro of the black strap to the splint	
Document the time of application and ensure this is communicated at handover	

T-POD® Stabilisation Device

Action	Check
Explain the procedure and obtain consent (unless the patient is unable to)	
Don appropriate PPE and undertake appropriate hand hygiene	
Check all the patient's clothing (including underwear) has been removed	
Ensure all parts are present and that the pulley system has been fully opened up and is not twisted	
As long as there are no other injuries that may be made worse, strap the feet together using a triangle bandage (or similar) in a figure of eight	
Locate the level of the greater trochanter	
Insert the belt under the legs, with the white side facing the patient	
Slide the belt up into position and confirm the centre of the binder is in line with the greater trochanters	
Cut the excess belt, leaving a 15–20 cm (6–8 in) gap over the centre of the pelvis	
Place the pulley system on the belt, ensuring that the Velcro is stuck down well	
Gently apply tension to the pull cord by pulling on the attached tab	
Once appropriate tension has been applied, wrap the excess pull cord around the vertical posts located next to the pulleys until the excess cord has been wrapped up sufficiently for the plastic tab to be conveniently stuck to the Velcro	
Stick the plastic tab down so it is secure	
Document the time of application and ensure this is communicated at handover	

Manual In-Line Stabilisation

Action	Check
Explain the procedure and obtain consent (unless the patient is unable to)	
Don appropriate PPE and undertake appropriate hand hygiene	
Advise the patient not to move their head	
Explain that you are going to hold their head to help keep it still	
Place yourself in a comfortable position behind the patient	
Place your hands either side of the head and over the mastoid process	
If the patient's head is not facing forward and the patient is conscious, ask them to slowly move their head into a neutral, in-line position[1]	
Maintain manual in-line stabilisation (MILS) until patient is fully immobilised or immobilisation is no longer required	
Document the procedure, including time it was undertaken and any complications	

Note:
1. Movement to the neutral position should cease if there is:
   a. Resistance to movement
   b. Neck muscle spasm
   c. Increased pain
   d. An increase in neurological deficit (numbness, tingling etc.).
   In any of these cases the neck should be immobilised in the position that it presents in.

Helmet Removal

Action	Check
If the patient is conscious, explain the procedure and obtain consent (unless the patient is unable to)	
Don appropriate PPE and undertake appropriate hand hygiene	
The clinician leading the procedure should verbalise the plan and ensure others involved are clear on the process and their roles	
One rescuer should position themselves at the head end and take a grip of the helmet	
From the side, a second rescuer should remove the face shield if present and release the chin strap/padding where possible. Remove EQRS padding, if present	
The second rescuer should take control of the head. Once in position with a firm grip, this rescuer should say 'I'm on'	
Rescuer one can now gently rock the helmet back and forth whilst pulling the sides of the helmet slightly apart and applying traction	
Once the helmet is approximately halfway off, rescuer one should stop moving the helmet and adjust their hands, so they have control of the neck and movement of the head through the helmet. Once they have control, they should say 'I'm on'	
Rescuer two should adjust their hands to ensure they have a good grip. Once in position, with a firm grip controlling the head and neck, rescuer two should declare 'I'm on'	
Rescuer one should continue to rock the helmet whilst applying traction until the head is released	
Set the helmet to one side ready to convey to hospital with the patient	
Rescuer one should now apply manual in-line stabilisation (MILS) and in a co-ordinated move lower the head to neutral alignment along with rescuer two[1]	
Document the procedure	

Note:
1. If any resistance is felt whilst lowering to neutral alignment then cease immediately and pad in the current position.

Cervical Collar – Adults

Action	Check
Explain the procedure to the patient and obtain consent (unless the patient is unable to)	
Don appropriate PPE and undertake appropriate hand hygiene	
Ensure you have the correct equipment and, where possible, three people available to apply the collar	
Ensure the head is in a neutral position	
Assign a rescuer to maintain manual in-line stabilisation (MILS)	
Size the collar	
Compare the distance measured with the space on the collar between the sizing line and the lower aspect of the plastic part of the collar body (not the foam)	
Adjust the collar to the appropriate size	
Engage locking pins	
Ensure chin piece has been flipped over	
Offer the front of the collar up to the patient's chin and chest and check sizing. Adjust if necessary	
Roll the collar to pre-form prior to application	
Slide the back part of the collar under the patient's neck until the Velcro can be seen appearing on the other side	
Position the chin piece under the chin	
While keeping the front of the collar in the correct position with one hand, attach the Velcro with your other hand to achieve a secure fit	
Maintain MILS until neck is fully immobilised	
Document the procedure and time it was completed	

Scoop Stretcher

Action	Check
If the patient is conscious, explain the procedure and obtain consent (unless the patient is unable to)	
Don appropriate PPE and undertake appropriate hand hygiene	
If indicated, ensure manual in-line stabilisation (MILS) is being applied and a cervical collar has been fitted	
Ensure that the patient is exposed appropriately, and any other equipment required has been gathered	
Place the scoop on the ground next to the patient so that the head is in line with the area that is designed to accommodate the head on the scoop stretcher	
Move the locking pins on either side of the stretcher to the upright position. Adjust the length of the stretcher by pulling on the foot section until the scoop stretcher is the desired length	
Move the locking pins to the downward position. Gently move the foot section up and down until it locks into place	
Separate the scoop stretcher by pressing the tabs on the Twin Safety Lock system at both the head and foot ends	
Ensure you have enough people to undertake the procedure. You will require people for each of the following: • MILS (if indicated) • Two people to undertake the roll • One person to insert the scoop stretcher. The team leader should brief everyone as to their role and the steps involved.	
Position rescuers for the procedure	
When all rescuers are ready, the clinician at the head end of the patient should issue the command: 'Ready, set, move.' On 'move', the clinicians should conduct a coordinated roll. Once completed, the scoop stretcher should be inserted under the patient	

Chapter 6 – *Trauma*

Action	Check
Once the scoop stretcher has been inserted, the patient should be lowered using the same 'Ready, set, move' command issued by the clinician at the head end of the patient	
Repeat the procedure on the other side	
Once both boards are in place, push the brackets of the Twin Safety Lock together until clicked into position. Start with the bracket at the head end	
Secure the patient to the stretcher by attaching the chest straps first. If possible, ask the patient to take a deep breath and hold it before tightening the chest straps	
Apply the hip strap and secure	
Apply the foot strap in a figure-of-eight configuration	
Secure the head using a system designed for use with a scoop stretcher	
Document the procedure	

Trauma

Vacuum Mattress

Action	Check
If the patient is conscious, explain the procedure and obtain consent (unless the patient is unable to)	
Don appropriate PPE and undertake appropriate hand hygiene	
Lay the vacuum mattress out on the floor. Check which end is the head end and extend all the buckles on the straps so they are fully open prior to placing the patient in the device	
Check the mattress has no leaks, by quickly removing the air and ensuring it does not rapidly lose its vacuum effect	
Prepare the patient by removing clothing as necessary and use a scoop stretcher to transfer them into the mattress	
With one person providing manual in-line stabilisation (MILS) of the cervical spine, one or two more clinicians should start to buckle up the straps, working from the chest down	
To tighten, two clinicians should apply equal opposing force to the buckle. While tightening the chest straps, ask the patient to take a deep breath in and hold it	
Secure the thigh strap (colour coded) and the two foot straps	
Another clinician should take control of the cervical spine from the side to release clinician providing MILS	
Once the hands on the sides of the head have been released, a device for immobilising the head can be inserted	
Form the vacuum mattress securely around the head blocks. Once the head is controlled from the sides through the mattress, the immobilisation of the forehead and chin can be released	
Check that the valve is securely in the closed position and attach the pump which has been set up to extract air	
With one person maintaining manual control of the head, another should pump the air out of the mattress. Any spare rescuers can help to gently form the body of the mattress to the patient	
Continue to remove air until the mattress becomes firm and can no longer be easily reshaped by hand	

Chapter 6 – *Trauma*

Action	Check
Check the straps; if any have become loose, retighten now	
Strap the head down using appropriate straps or tape	
If the patient subsequently requires removing from the mattress, a scoop stretcher should be used	
Document the procedure	

Cardiac Arrest: An Advisory Note

Checklists for managing cardiac arrest scenarios, such as those involving basic or advanced life support, have been intentionally omitted from this book. These situations usually require a more nuanced and dynamic approach to assessment than a simple tick-box format can provide.

Cardiac arrest management is made up of a number of individual procedures (for example airway insertion and bag-valve-mask ventilation) but the judgement required to bring all of these procedures together to provide overall effective care, which often needs to be modified to fit the precise situation encountered, is beyond the scope of a single checklist of purely objective steps. Cardiac arrest assessment needs to consider both objective and subjective aspects including areas such as leadership techniques, communication and forward planning.

Education providers will develop their own methodologies for the more complex assessment of competence in cardiac arrest management, tailored to their programmes and aligned with current national best practice and guidelines.

Infection Prevention and Control

Hand Hygiene with Soap and Running Water

Action	Check
Wet hands with water	
Apply enough soap to cover all areas	
Rub hands palm to palm	
Rub your right palm over the back of the left hand with interlaced fingers and vice versa	
Rub palm to palm with fingers interlaced	
Rub the backs of your fingers to opposing palms with fingers interlocked	
Rub the left thumb in your right palm in a rotational motion and vice versa	
Clasp the fingers of your right hand in your left palm, and rub in a rotational motion, backwards and forwards, and vice versa	
Rinse hands with water	
Dry thoroughly with a disposable towel	
Where possible, use your elbows to turn off taps. If this is not possible, use a towel to turn off taps	

Hand Hygiene with Alcohol-Based Hand Rub

Action	Check
Apply a palmful of the product into a cupped hand and cover all surfaces	
Rub hands palm to palm	
Rub your right palm over the back of the left hand with interlaced fingers and vice versa	
Rub palm to palm with fingers interlaced	
Rub the backs of your fingers to opposing palms with fingers interlocked	
Rub the left thumb in your right palm in a rotational motion and vice versa	
Clasp the fingers of your right hand in your left palm, and rub in a rotational motion, backwards and forwards, and vice versa	
Once dry, your hands are safe	

Donning PPE for Standard Infection Prevention Control

Action	Check
Ensure you have the required PPE in the correct sizes: • Disposable apron • Surgical face mask • Disposable gloves • Eye protection (goggles or visor, if required) • Alcohol-based hand rub	
Remove any items from the pockets of clothing, tie back hair and remove jewellery	
Perform hand hygiene using an alcohol-based hand rub	
Place head through beck loop of apron and fasten behind your back	
Put on face mask	
Apply eye protection and adjust to ensure a secure fit	
Put on disposable gloves	

Donning PPE for Aerosol Generating Procedures

Action	Check
Ensure you have the required PPE in the correct sizes: • Disposable coveralls • Respiratory protection • Disposable gloves • Eye protection (goggles or visor)	
Remove any items from the pockets of clothing, tie back hair and remove jewellery	
Don coveralls	
Apply an appropriate respirator, either a mask or powered hood	
Apply eye protection and adjust as required	
Put on disposable gloves, ensuring that cuff of glove covers the cuff of the coveralls	

Doffing PPE for Standard Infection Prevention Control

Action	Check
Plan your movements	
Grasp the outside of a glove with the opposite gloved hand and peel off	
Slide a finger from the ungloved hand under the wrist of the gloved hand, hook the glove and peel it off	
Dispose of both gloves into a clinical waste bag	
Perform hand hygiene using an alcohol-based hand rub	
Remove the disposable apron and dispose	
Remove eye protection and dispose	
Perform hand hygiene using an alcohol-based hand rub	
Once outside of the ambulance or patient's immediate environment, remove the surgical face mask and dispose	
Perform hand hygiene with soap and water if available; if not, use an alcohol-based hand rub	

Infection Prevention and Control

Doffing PPE for Aerosol Generating Procedures

Action	Check
Move away from the patient	
Don appropriate PPE and undertake appropriate hand hygiene	
Grasp the outside of a glove with the opposite gloved hand and peel off	
Slide a finger from the ungloved hand under the wrist of the gloved hand, hook the glove and peel it off	
Perform hand hygiene using an alcohol-based hand rub	
Remove coveralls from top to bottom and dispose	
Perform hand hygiene using an alcohol-based hand rub	
Remove eye protection and dispose	
Perform hand hygiene using an alcohol-based hand rub	
Remove the respirator and dispose	
Perform hand hygiene with soap and water if available; if not, use an alcohol-based hand rub